This Pain Tracker
Belongs to

_____

_____

_____

DEDICATION

This Pain Journal Log Book is dedicated to all the pain sufferers out there who want to track their pain and document their findings in the process.

You are my inspiration for producing books and I'm honored to be a part of keeping all of your Chronic Pain notes and records organized.

This journal notebook will help you record your details about your pain.

Thoughtfully put together with these sections to record: Date, Weather Conditions, Symptoms, Sleep, Fatigue, Pain, Brain Fog, Mood, Body Diagram, Stress At Home, Stress At Work, Color Code Pain Level, Food Tracker, Medication, and Notes.

How To Use This Book:

The purpose of this book is to keep all of your Pain notes all in one place. It will help keep you organized.

This Pain Journal will allow you to accurately document every detail about your symptoms and pain level. It's a great way to chart your course through dealing with your pain.

Here are examples of the prompts for you to fill in and write about your experience in this book:

1. Date, Weather, Temp, Conditions, Humidity - Record the weather to see if there are correlations with your pain.
2. My Symptoms - List your symptom or symptoms.
3. How Well Did You Sleep - Rate on a scale of 1-10?
4. How Was Your Pain Today - Rate the severity of your pain on a scale of 1-10.
5. How Was Your Fatigue Today - Rate on a scale of 1-10?
6. How Was Your Brain Fog Today - Rate on a scale of 1-10?
7. How Was Your Mood Today - Rate on a scale of 1-10?
8. Body Diagram - To track the location of your pain.
9. Stress Levels Assessment At Work - Rate on a scale of 1-10.
10. Stress Levels Assessment At Home - Rate on a scale of 1-10.
11. Code & Color In Your Pain Level Sections - Monitor your pain by coloring in the description of your pain (Shooting, stabbing, burning, numbness, aching, pins & needles, other).
12. Food Tracker - List what you had for breakfast, lunch, dinner, snacks & drinks.
13. Medication - List your medications for the day.
14. Supplements & Vitamins - List your supplements & vitamins for the day.
15. Notes - For writing any other important information such as other health or medical issues, migraine, headaches or headache, duration of pain, any illness, how you got relief, well check-ups at the doctors.

Enjoy!

Daily Chronic Pain Tracker

Date:

Weather
Temp:
Condition:
Humidity:

My Symptoms
_____
_____
_____

How well did you sleep?
1 2 3 4 5 6 7 8 9 10

How was your pain today?
1 2 3 4 5 6 7 8 9 10

How was your fatigue today?
1 2 3 4 5 6 7 8 9 10

How was your brain fog today?
1 2 3 4 5 6 7 8 9 10

How was your mood today?
1 2 3 4 5 6 7 8 9 10

Food Tracker
Breakfast _____
_____
_____

Lunch _____
_____

Dinner _____
_____
_____
_____

Snacks/Drinks _____
_____

Code & Color in your Pain

☐ *Shooting*
☐ *Stabbing*
☐ *Burning*
☐ *Numbness*
☐ *Aching*
☐ *Pins & Needles*
☐ *Other*

NOTES
_____
_____
_____
_____
_____
_____
_____
_____
_____
_____
_____
_____

Stress levels at home
1 2 3 4 5
6 7 8 9 10

Stress levels at work
1 2 3 4 5
6 7 8 9 10

Medication

Supplements

Vitamins

Daily Chronic Pain Tracker

Date:

Weather
Temp:
Condition:
Humidity:

My Symptoms
_____
_____
_____
_____

How well did you sleep?
1 2 3 4 5 6 7 8 9 10

How was your pain today?
1 2 3 4 5 6 7 8 9 10

How was your fatigue today?
1 2 3 4 5 6 7 8 9 10

How was your brain fog today?
1 2 3 4 5 6 7 8 9 10

How was your mood today?
1 2 3 4 5 6 7 8 9 10

Food Tracker
Breakfast _____
_____
_____

Lunch _____
_____
_____

Dinner _____
_____
_____
_____

Snacks/Drinks
_____
_____
_____

Code & Color in your Pain

[ ] Shooting
[ ] Stabbing
[ ] Burning
[ ] Numbness
[ ] Aching
[ ] Pins & Needles
[ ] Other

Medication

Supplements

Vitamins

NOTES
_____
_____
_____
_____
_____
_____
_____
_____
_____
_____
_____

Stress levels at home
1 2 3 4 5
6 7 8 9 10

Stress levels at work
1 2 3 4 5
6 7 8 9 10

Daily Chronic Pain Tracker

Date:

Weather
Temp:
Condition:
Humidity:

My Symptoms
_____
_____
_____
_____

How well did you sleep?
1 2 3 4 5 6 7 8 9 10

How was your pain today?
1 2 3 4 5 6 7 8 9 10

How was your fatigue today?
1 2 3 4 5 6 7 8 9 10

How was your brain fog today?
1 2 3 4 5 6 7 8 9 10

How was your mood today?
1 2 3 4 5 6 7 8 9 10

Food Tracker
Breakfast
_____
_____
_____

Lunch
_____
_____
_____

Dinner
_____
_____
_____
_____

Snacks/Drinks
_____
_____
_____

Code & Color in your Pain

☐	Shooting
☐	Stabbing
☐	Burning
☐	Numbness
☐	Aching
☐	Pins & Needles
☐	Other

Medication

Supplements

Vitamins

NOTES
_____
_____
_____
_____
_____
_____
_____
_____
_____
_____
_____
_____
_____

Stress levels at home
1 2 3 4 5
6 7 8 9 10

Stress levels at work
1 2 3 4 5
6 7 8 9 10

Daily Chronic Pain Tracker

Date:

Weather
Temp:
Condition:
Humidity:

My Symptoms
_____
_____
_____
_____

How well did you sleep?
1 2 3 4 5 6 7 8 9 10

How was your pain today?
1 2 3 4 5 6 7 8 9 10

How was your fatigue today?
1 2 3 4 5 6 7 8 9 10

How was your brain fog today?
1 2 3 4 5 6 7 8 9 10

How was your mood today?
1 2 3 4 5 6 7 8 9 10

Food Tracker
Breakfast _____
_____
_____

Lunch _____
_____
_____

Dinner _____
_____
_____
_____

Snacks/Drinks
_____
_____

Code & Color in your Pain

[ ] Shooting _____
[ ] Stabbing _____
[ ] Burning
[ ] Numbness
[ ] Aching
[ ] Pins & Needles
[ ] Other

Medication

NOTES
_____
_____
_____
_____
_____
_____
_____
_____
_____
_____
_____
_____
_____

Supplements

Vitamins

Stress levels at home
1 2 3 4 5
6 7 8 9 10

Stress levels at work
1 2 3 4 5
6 7 8 9 10

Daily Chronic Pain Tracker

Date:

Weather
Temp:
Condition:
Humidity:

My Symptoms
_____
_____
_____
_____

How well did you sleep?
1 2 3 4 5 6 7 8 9 10

How was your pain today?
1 2 3 4 5 6 7 8 9 10

How was your fatigue today?
1 2 3 4 5 6 7 8 9 10

How was your brain fog today?
1 2 3 4 5 6 7 8 9 10

How was your mood today?
1 2 3 4 5 6 7 8 9 10

Food Tracker
Breakfast
_____
_____
_____

Lunch
_____
_____
_____

Dinner
_____
_____
_____
_____

Snacks/Drinks
_____
_____

Code & Color in your Pain

- [ ] Shooting _____
- [ ] Stabbing _____
- [ ] Burning
- [ ] Numbness
- [ ] Aching
- [ ] Pins & Needles
- [ ] Other

Medication

NOTES

_____
_____
_____
_____
_____
_____
_____
_____
_____
_____
_____
_____
_____
_____
_____

Supplements

Vitamins

Stress levels at home
1 2 3 4 5
6 7 8 9 10

Stress levels at work
1 2 3 4 5
6 7 8 9 10

Daily Chronic Pain Tracker

Date:

Weather

Temp:

Condition:

Humidity:

My Symptoms

_____
_____
_____
_____

How well did you sleep?
1 2 3 4 5 6 7 8 9 10

How was your pain today?
1 2 3 4 5 6 7 8 9 10

How was your fatigue today?
1 2 3 4 5 6 7 8 9 10

How was your brain fog today?
1 2 3 4 5 6 7 8 9 10

How was your mood today?
1 2 3 4 5 6 7 8 9 10

Food Tracker

Breakfast _____
_____
_____

Lunch _____
_____
_____

Dinner _____
_____
_____
_____

Snacks/Drinks
_____
_____

Code & Color
in your Pain

[ ] Shooting _____

[ ] Stabbing _____

[ ] Burning

[ ] Numbness

[ ] Aching

[ ] Pins & Needles

[ ] Other

Medication

Supplements

Vitamins

NOTES
_____
_____
_____
_____
_____
_____
_____
_____
_____
_____
_____
_____

Stress levels at home
1 2 3 4 5
6 7 8 9 10

Stress levels at work
1 2 3 4 5
6 7 8 9 10

Daily Chronic Pain Tracker

Date:

Weather
Temp:
Condition:
Humidity:

My Symptoms
_____
_____
_____
_____

How well did you sleep?
1 2 3 4 5 6 7 8 9 10

How was your pain today?
1 2 3 4 5 6 7 8 9 10

How was your fatigue today?
1 2 3 4 5 6 7 8 9 10

How was your brain fog today?
1 2 3 4 5 6 7 8 9 10

How was your mood today?
1 2 3 4 5 6 7 8 9 10

Food Tracker
Breakfast
_____
_____
_____
Lunch _____
_____
_____
Dinner _____
_____
_____
_____
_____

Snacks/Drinks
_____
_____

Code & Color in your Pain

[ ] Shooting
[ ] Stabbing
[ ] Burning
[ ] Numbness
[ ] Aching
[ ] Pins & Needles
[ ] Other

Medication
|
|
|
Supplements
|
|
|
Vitamins
|
|

NOTES
_____
_____
_____
_____
_____
_____
_____
_____
_____
_____
_____

Stress levels at home
1 2 3 4 5
6 7 8 9 10

Stress levels at work
1 2 3 4 5
6 7 8 9 10

Daily Chronic Pain Tracker

Date:

Weather
Temp:
Condition:
Humidity:

My Symptoms
_____
_____
_____
_____

How well did you sleep?
1 2 3 4 5 6 7 8 9 10

How was your pain today?
1 2 3 4 5 6 7 8 9 10

How was your fatigue today?
1 2 3 4 5 6 7 8 9 10

How was your brain fog today?
1 2 3 4 5 6 7 8 9 10

How was your mood today?
1 2 3 4 5 6 7 8 9 10

Food Tracker

Breakfast _____

_____

Lunch _____

_____

Dinner _____

_____

Snacks/Drinks _____

_____

Code & Color in your Pain

☐	Shooting
☐	Stabbing
☐	Burning
☐	Numbness
☐	Aching
☐	Pins & Needles
☐	Other

Medication

Supplements

Vitamins

NOTES
_____
_____
_____
_____
_____
_____
_____
_____
_____
_____
_____

Stress levels at home
1 2 3 4 5
6 7 8 9 10

Stress levels at work
1 2 3 4 5
6 7 8 9 10

Daily Chronic Pain Tracker

Date:

Weather
Temp:
Condition:
Humidity:

My Symptoms
_____
_____
_____
_____

How well did you sleep?
1 2 3 4 5 6 7 8 9 10

How was your pain today?
1 2 3 4 5 6 7 8 9 10

How was your fatigue today?
1 2 3 4 5 6 7 8 9 10

How was your brain fog today?
1 2 3 4 5 6 7 8 9 10

How was your mood today?
1 2 3 4 5 6 7 8 9 10

Food Tracker
Breakfast
_____
_____
_____

Lunch
_____
_____
_____

Dinner
_____
_____
_____
_____

Snacks/Drinks
_____
_____

Code & Color in your Pain

[ ] Shooting
[ ] Stabbing
[ ] Burning
[ ] Numbness
[ ] Aching
[ ] Pins & Needles
[ ] Other

Medication

Supplements

Vitamins

NOTES
_____
_____
_____
_____
_____
_____
_____
_____
_____
_____
_____
_____

Stress levels at home
1 2 3 4 5
6 7 8 9 10

Stress levels at work
1 2 3 4 5
6 7 8 9 10

Daily Chronic Pain Tracker

Date:

Weather

Temp:

Condition:

Humidity:

My Symptoms

_____
_____
_____
_____

How well did you sleep?
1 2 3 4 5 6 7 8 9 10

How was your pain today?
1 2 3 4 5 6 7 8 9 10

How was your fatigue today?
1 2 3 4 5 6 7 8 9 10

How was your brain fog today?
1 2 3 4 5 6 7 8 9 10

How was your mood today?
1 2 3 4 5 6 7 8 9 10

Food Tracker

Breakfast _____
_____
_____
_____

Lunch _____
_____
_____

Dinner _____
_____
_____
_____
_____

Snacks/Drinks
_____
_____

Code & Color in your Pain

[ ] Shooting _____

[ ] Stabbing _____

[ ] Burning

[ ] Numbness

[ ] Aching

[ ] Pins & Needles

[ ] Other

Medication

NOTES
_____
_____
_____
_____
_____
_____
_____
_____
_____
_____
_____
_____
_____

Supplements

Vitamins

Stress levels at home

1 2 3 4 5
6 7 8 9 10

Stress levels at work

1 2 3 4 5
6 7 8 9 10

Daily Chronic Pain Tracker

Date:

Weather
Temp:
Condition:
Humidity:

My Symptoms
_____
_____
_____
_____

How well did you sleep?
1 2 3 4 5 6 7 8 9 10

How was your pain today?
1 2 3 4 5 6 7 8 9 10

How was your fatigue today?
1 2 3 4 5 6 7 8 9 10

How was your brain fog today?
1 2 3 4 5 6 7 8 9 10

How was your mood today?
1 2 3 4 5 6 7 8 9 10

Food Tracker

Breakfast
_____
_____
_____

Lunch
_____
_____
_____

Dinner
_____
_____
_____
_____

Snacks/Drinks
_____
_____
_____

Code & Color in your Pain

[ ] Shooting
[ ] Stabbing
[ ] Burning
[ ] Numbness
[ ] Aching
[ ] Pins & Needles
[ ] Other

Medication

NOTES
_____
_____
_____
_____
_____
_____
_____

Stress levels at home
1 2 3 4 5
6 7 8 9 10

Stress levels at work
1 2 3 4 5
6 7 8 9 10

_____
_____
_____
_____
_____

Supplements

Vitamins

Daily Chronic Pain Tracker

Date:

Weather
Temp:
Condition:
Humidity:

My Symptoms
_____
_____
_____
_____

How well did you sleep?
1 2 3 4 5 6 7 8 9 10

How was your pain today?
1 2 3 4 5 6 7 8 9 10

How was your fatigue today?
1 2 3 4 5 6 7 8 9 10

How was your brain fog today?
1 2 3 4 5 6 7 8 9 10

How was your mood today?
1 2 3 4 5 6 7 8 9 10

Food Tracker
Breakfast _____
_____
_____
_____

Lunch _____
_____
_____

Dinner _____
_____
_____
_____
_____

Snacks/Drinks
_____
_____
_____

Code & Color in your Pain

[ ] Shooting
[ ] Stabbing
[ ] Burning
[ ] Numbness
[ ] Aching
[ ] Pins & Needles
[ ] Other

Medication

Supplements

Vitamins

NOTES
_____
_____
_____
_____
_____
_____
_____
_____
_____
_____
_____
_____
_____
_____

Stress levels at home
1 2 3 4 5
6 7 8 9 10

Stress levels at work
1 2 3 4 5
6 7 8 9 10

Daily Chronic Pain Tracker

Date:

Weather
Temp:
Condition:
Humidity:

My Symptoms
_____
_____
_____
_____

How well did you sleep?
1 2 3 4 5 6 7 8 9 10

How was your pain today?
1 2 3 4 5 6 7 8 9 10

How was your fatigue today?
1 2 3 4 5 6 7 8 9 10

How was your brain fog today?
1 2 3 4 5 6 7 8 9 10

How was your mood today?
1 2 3 4 5 6 7 8 9 10

Food Tracker
Breakfast _____
_____
_____
Lunch _____
_____
_____
Dinner _____
_____
_____
_____

**Code & Color
in your Pain**

[ ] Shooting
[ ] Stabbing
[ ] Burning
[ ] Numbness
[ ] Aching
[ ] Pins & Needles
[ ] Other

Snacks/Drinks
_____
_____

Medication

NOTES
_____
_____
_____
_____
_____
_____
_____
_____
_____
_____
_____
_____
_____

Supplements

Vitamins

Stress levels at home
1 2 3 4 5
6 7 8 9 10

Stress levels at work
1 2 3 4 5
6 7 8 9 10

Daily Chronic Pain Tracker

Date:

Weather
Temp:
Condition:
Humidity:

My Symptoms
_____
_____
_____
_____

How well did you sleep?
1 2 3 4 5 6 7 8 9 10

How was your pain today?
1 2 3 4 5 6 7 8 9 10

How was your fatigue today?
1 2 3 4 5 6 7 8 9 10

How was your brain fog today?
1 2 3 4 5 6 7 8 9 10

How was your mood today?
1 2 3 4 5 6 7 8 9 10

Food Tracker
Breakfast _____
_____
_____
Lunch _____
_____
_____
Dinner _____
_____
_____
_____

Snacks/Drinks
_____
_____

Code & Color in your Pain

[ ]	Shooting
[ ]	Stabbing
[ ]	Burning
[ ]	Numbness
[ ]	Aching
[ ]	Pins & Needles
[ ]	Other

Medication

Supplements

Vitamins

NOTES
_____
_____
_____
_____
_____
_____
_____
_____
_____
_____
_____
_____
_____

Stress levels at home
1 2 3 4 5
6 7 8 9 10

Stress levels at work
1 2 3 4 5
6 7 8 9 10

Daily Chronic Pain Tracker

Date:

Weather
Temp:
Condition:
Humidity:

My Symptoms
—————————
—————————
—————————

How well did you sleep?
1 2 3 4 5 6 7 8 9 10

How was your pain today?
1 2 3 4 5 6 7 8 9 10

How was your fatigue today?
1 2 3 4 5 6 7 8 9 10

How was your brain fog today?
1 2 3 4 5 6 7 8 9 10

How was your mood today?
1 2 3 4 5 6 7 8 9 10

Food Tracker
Breakfast ———
—————————
—————————
—————————
Lunch ————
—————————
—————————
—————————
Dinner ———
—————————
—————————
—————————
—————————

Snacks/Drinks
—————————
—————————

Code & Color in your Pain

[ ] Shooting
[ ] Stabbing
[ ] Burning
[ ] Numbness
[ ] Aching
[ ] Pins & Needles
[ ] Other

NOTES
—————————
—————————
—————————
—————————
—————————
—————————
—————————
—————————
—————————
—————————
—————————
—————————

Stress levels at home
1 2 3 4 5
6 7 8 9 10

Stress levels at work
1 2 3 4 5
6 7 8 9 10

Medication

Supplements

Vitamins

Daily Chronic Pain Tracker

Date:

Weather
Temp:
Condition:
Humidity:

My Symptoms
_____
_____
_____
_____

How well did you sleep?
1 2 3 4 5 6 7 8 9 10

How was your pain today?
1 2 3 4 5 6 7 8 9 10

How was your fatigue today?
1 2 3 4 5 6 7 8 9 10

How was your brain fog today?
1 2 3 4 5 6 7 8 9 10

How was your mood today?
1 2 3 4 5 6 7 8 9 10

Food Tracker
Breakfast
_____
_____
_____

Lunch
_____
_____
_____

Dinner
_____
_____
_____
_____

Snacks/Drinks
_____
_____
_____

Code & Color in your Pain

[ ] *Shooting*
[ ] *Stabbing*
[ ] *Burning*
[ ] *Numbness*
[ ] *Aching*
[ ] *Pins & Needles*
[ ] *Other*

Medication

Supplements

Vitamins

NOTES
_____
_____
_____
_____
_____
_____
_____
_____
_____
_____
_____
_____
_____
_____

Stress levels at home
1 2 3 4 5
6 7 8 9 10

Stress levels at work
1 2 3 4 5
6 7 8 9 10

Daily Chronic Pain Tracker

Date:

Weather
Temp:
Condition:
Humidity:

My Symptoms
_____
_____
_____
_____

How well did you sleep?
1 2 3 4 5 6 7 8 9 10

How was your pain today?
1 2 3 4 5 6 7 8 9 10

How was your fatigue today?
1 2 3 4 5 6 7 8 9 10

How was your brain fog today?
1 2 3 4 5 6 7 8 9 10

How was your mood today?
1 2 3 4 5 6 7 8 9 10

Code & Color in your Pain

☐	Shooting
☐	Stabbing
☐	Burning
☐	Numbness
☐	Aching
☐	Pins & Needles
☐	Other

NOTES
_____
_____
_____
_____
_____
_____
_____
_____
_____
_____
_____
_____

Stress levels at home
1 2 3 4 5
6 7 8 9 10

Stress levels at work
1 2 3 4 5
6 7 8 9 10

Food Tracker

Breakfast
_____
_____
_____

Lunch
_____
_____
_____

Dinner
_____
_____
_____

Snacks/Drinks
_____
_____

Medication

Supplements

Vitamins

Daily Chronic Pain Tracker

Date:

Weather
Temp:
Condition:
Humidity:

My Symptoms
_____
_____
_____
_____

How well did you sleep?
1 2 3 4 5 6 7 8 9 10

How was your pain today?
1 2 3 4 5 6 7 8 9 10

How was your fatigue today?
1 2 3 4 5 6 7 8 9 10

How was your brain fog today?
1 2 3 4 5 6 7 8 9 10

How was your mood today?
1 2 3 4 5 6 7 8 9 10

Food Tracker
Breakfast _____
_____
_____
Lunch _____
_____
_____
Dinner _____
_____
_____
_____
Snacks/Drinks _____
_____
_____

Code & Color in your Pain

[ ] *Shooting*
[ ] *Stabbing*
[ ] *Burning*
[ ] *Numbness*
[ ] *Aching*
[ ] *Pins & Needles*
[ ] *Other*

Medication

Supplements

Vitamins

NOTES
_____
_____
_____
_____
_____
_____
_____
_____
_____
_____
_____

Stress levels at home
1 2 3 4 5
6 7 8 9 10

Stress levels at work
1 2 3 4 5
6 7 8 9 10

Daily Chronic Pain Tracker

Date:

Weather
Temp:
Condition:
Humidity:

My Symptoms
_____
_____
_____
_____

How well did you sleep?
1 2 3 4 5 6 7 8 9 10

How was your pain today?
1 2 3 4 5 6 7 8 9 10

How was your fatigue today?
1 2 3 4 5 6 7 8 9 10

How was your brain fog today?
1 2 3 4 5 6 7 8 9 10

How was your mood today?
1 2 3 4 5 6 7 8 9 10

Food Tracker
Breakfast
_____
_____
_____

Lunch
_____
_____
_____

Dinner
_____
_____
_____
_____
_____

Snacks/Drinks
_____
_____

Code & Color in your Pain

[ ]	Shooting
[ ]	Stabbing
[ ]	Burning
[ ]	Numbness
[ ]	Aching
[ ]	Pins & Needles
[ ]	Other

NOTES
_____
_____
_____
_____
_____
_____
_____
_____
_____
_____
_____
_____
_____

Medication

Supplements

Vitamins

Stress levels at home
1 2 3 4 5
6 7 8 9 10

Stress levels at work
1 2 3 4 5
6 7 8 9 10

Daily Chronic Pain Tracker

Date:

Weather
Temp:
Condition:
Humidity:

My Symptoms
_____
_____
_____
_____

How well did you sleep?
1 2 3 4 5 6 7 8 9 10

How was your pain today?
1 2 3 4 5 6 7 8 9 10

How was your fatigue today?
1 2 3 4 5 6 7 8 9 10

How was your brain fog today?
1 2 3 4 5 6 7 8 9 10

How was your mood today?
1 2 3 4 5 6 7 8 9 10

Food Tracker
Breakfast _____
_____
_____
_____

Lunch _____
_____
_____

Dinner _____
_____
_____
_____
_____

Snacks/Drinks
_____
_____
_____

Code & Color in your Pain

☐ *Shooting*
☐ *Stabbing*
☐ *Burning*
☐ *Numbness*
☐ *Aching*
☐ *Pins & Needles*
☐ *Other*

NOTES
_____
_____
_____
_____
_____
_____
_____
_____
_____
_____
_____
_____
_____
_____

Stress levels at home
1 2 3 4 5
6 7 8 9 10

Stress levels at work
1 2 3 4 5
6 7 8 9 10

Medication

Supplements

Vitamins

Daily Chronic Pain Tracker

Date:

Weather

Temp:

Condition:

Humidity:

My Symptoms
_____
_____
_____
_____

How well did you sleep?
1 2 3 4 5 6 7 8 9 10

How was your pain today?
1 2 3 4 5 6 7 8 9 10

How was your fatigue today?
1 2 3 4 5 6 7 8 9 10

How was your brain fog today?
1 2 3 4 5 6 7 8 9 10

How was your mood today?
1 2 3 4 5 6 7 8 9 10

Food Tracker
Breakfast _____
_____
_____

Lunch _____
_____
_____

Dinner _____
_____
_____
_____

Snacks/Drinks _____
_____
_____

Code & Color in your Pain

☐	Shooting
☐	Stabbing
☐	Burning
☐	Numbness
☐	Aching
☐	Pins & Needles
☐	Other

NOTES
_____
_____
_____
_____
_____
_____
_____
_____
_____
_____

Medication

Supplements

Vitamins

Stress levels at home

1 2 3 4 5
6 7 8 9 10

Stress levels at work

1 2 3 4 5
6 7 8 9 10

Daily Chronic Pain Tracker

Date:

Weather
Temp:
Condition:
Humidity:

My Symptoms
_____
_____
_____
_____

How well did you sleep?
1 2 3 4 5 6 7 8 9 10

How was your pain today?
1 2 3 4 5 6 7 8 9 10

How was your fatigue today?
1 2 3 4 5 6 7 8 9 10

How was your brain fog today?
1 2 3 4 5 6 7 8 9 10

How was your mood today?
1 2 3 4 5 6 7 8 9 10

Food Tracker
Breakfast _____
_____
_____
_____

Lunch _____
_____
_____
_____

Dinner _____
_____
_____
_____
_____

Snacks/Drinks _____
_____
_____

Code & Color in your Pain

[ ] Shooting _____
[ ] Stabbing _____
[ ] Burning
[ ] Numbness
[ ] Aching
[ ] Pins & Needles
[ ] Other

Medication

NOTES
_____
_____
_____
_____
_____
_____
_____
_____
_____
_____
_____
_____
_____

Supplements

Vitamins

Stress levels at home
1 2 3 4 5
6 7 8 9 10

Stress levels at work
1 2 3 4 5
6 7 8 9 10

Daily Chronic Pain Tracker

Date:

Weather
Temp:
Condition:
Humidity:

My Symptoms
_____
_____
_____
_____

How well did you sleep?
1 2 3 4 5 6 7 8 9 10

How was your pain today?
1 2 3 4 5 6 7 8 9 10

How was your fatigue today?
1 2 3 4 5 6 7 8 9 10

How was your brain fog today?
1 2 3 4 5 6 7 8 9 10

How was your mood today?
1 2 3 4 5 6 7 8 9 10

Food Tracker
Breakfast _____
_____
_____
_____

Lunch _____
_____
_____
_____

Dinner _____
_____
_____
_____

Code & Color in your Pain

☐	*Shooting*
☐	*Stabbing*
☐	*Burning*
☐	*Numbness*
☐	*Aching*
☐	*Pins & Needles*
☐	*Other*

Snacks/Drinks _____
_____

Medication

Supplements

Vitamins

NOTES
_____
_____
_____
_____
_____
_____
_____
_____
_____
_____
_____

Stress levels at home
1 2 3 4 5
6 7 8 9 10

Stress levels at work
1 2 3 4 5
6 7 8 9 10

Daily Chronic Pain Tracker

Date:

Weather
Temp:
Condition:
Humidity:

My Symptoms
_____
_____
_____
_____

How well did you sleep?
1 2 3 4 5 6 7 8 9 10

How was your pain today?
1 2 3 4 5 6 7 8 9 10

How was your fatigue today?
1 2 3 4 5 6 7 8 9 10

How was your brain fog today?
1 2 3 4 5 6 7 8 9 10

How was your mood today?
1 2 3 4 5 6 7 8 9 10

Food Tracker
Breakfast
_____
_____
_____

Lunch
_____
_____
_____

Dinner
_____
_____
_____
_____

Snacks/Drinks
_____
_____
_____

Code & Color in your Pain

☐ Shooting
☐ Stabbing
☐ Burning
☐ Numbness
☐ Aching
☐ Pins & Needles
☐ Other

Medication

NOTES
_____
_____
_____
_____
_____
_____
_____
_____
_____
_____
_____
_____
_____

Supplements

Vitamins

Stress levels at home
1 2 3 4 5
6 7 8 9 10

Stress levels at work
1 2 3 4 5
6 7 8 9 10

Daily Chronic Pain Tracker

Date:

Weather
Temp:
Condition:
Humidity:

My Symptoms
_____
_____
_____
_____

How well did you sleep?
1 2 3 4 5 6 7 8 9 10

How was your pain today?
1 2 3 4 5 6 7 8 9 10

How was your fatigue today?
1 2 3 4 5 6 7 8 9 10

How was your brain fog today?
1 2 3 4 5 6 7 8 9 10

How was your mood today?
1 2 3 4 5 6 7 8 9 10

Food Tracker
Breakfast
_____
_____
_____

Lunch
_____
_____
_____

Dinner
_____
_____
_____
_____

Snacks/Drinks
_____
_____
_____

Code & Color in your Pain

[ ] Shooting
[ ] Stabbing
[ ] Burning
[ ] Numbness
[ ] Aching
[ ] Pins & Needles
[ ] Other

Medication

Supplements

Vitamins

NOTES
_____
_____
_____
_____
_____
_____
_____
_____
_____
_____
_____
_____

Stress levels at home
1 2 3 4 5
6 7 8 9 10

Stress levels at work
1 2 3 4 5
6 7 8 9 10

Daily Chronic Pain Tracker

Date:

Weather
Temp:
Condition:
Humidity:

My Symptoms
_____
_____
_____
_____

How well did you sleep?
1 2 3 4 5 6 7 8 9 10

How was your pain today?
1 2 3 4 5 6 7 8 9 10

How was your fatigue today?
1 2 3 4 5 6 7 8 9 10

How was your brain fog today?
1 2 3 4 5 6 7 8 9 10

How was your mood today?
1 2 3 4 5 6 7 8 9 10

Food Tracker
Breakfast
_____
_____

Lunch
_____
_____

Dinner
_____
_____
_____

Snacks/Drinks
_____
_____

Code & Color in your Pain

☐	Shooting
☐	Stabbing
☐	Burning
☐	Numbness
☐	Aching
☐	Pins & Needles
☐	Other

Medication

Supplements

Vitamins

NOTES
_____
_____
_____
_____
_____
_____
_____
_____
_____
_____
_____
_____

Stress levels at home
1 2 3 4 5
6 7 8 9 10

Stress levels at work
1 2 3 4 5
6 7 8 9 10

Daily Chronic Pain Tracker

Date:

Weather
Temp:
Condition:
Humidity:

My Symptoms
_____
_____
_____
_____

How well did you sleep?
1 2 3 4 5 6 7 8 9 10

How was your pain today?
1 2 3 4 5 6 7 8 9 10

How was your fatigue today?
1 2 3 4 5 6 7 8 9 10

How was your brain fog today?
1 2 3 4 5 6 7 8 9 10

How was your mood today?
1 2 3 4 5 6 7 8 9 10

Food Tracker
Breakfast
_____
_____
_____

Lunch
_____
_____
_____

Dinner
_____
_____
_____
_____

Code & Color
in your Pain

Snacks/Drinks
_____
_____
_____

[ ] Shooting
[ ] Stabbing
[ ] Burning
[ ] Numbness
[ ] Aching
[ ] Pins & Needles
[ ] Other

Medication

NOTES
_____
_____
_____
_____
_____
_____
_____
_____
_____
_____
_____

Supplements

Stress levels at home
1 2 3 4 5
6 7 8 9 10

Stress levels at work
1 2 3 4 5
6 7 8 9 10

Vitamins

Daily Chronic Pain Tracker

Date:

Weather
Temp:
Condition:
Humidity:

My Symptoms
_____
_____
_____
_____

How well did you sleep?
1 2 3 4 5 6 7 8 9 10

How was your pain today?
1 2 3 4 5 6 7 8 9 10

How was your fatigue today?
1 2 3 4 5 6 7 8 9 10

How was your brain fog today?
1 2 3 4 5 6 7 8 9 10

How was your mood today?
1 2 3 4 5 6 7 8 9 10

Food Tracker
Breakfast
_____
_____

Lunch
_____
_____
_____

Dinner
_____
_____
_____

Snacks/Drinks
_____
_____

Code & Color in your Pain

[ ]	Shooting
[ ]	Stabbing
[ ]	Burning
[ ]	Numbness
[ ]	Aching
[ ]	Pins & Needles
[ ]	Other

Medication

Supplements

Vitamins

NOTES
_____
_____
_____
_____
_____
_____
_____
_____
_____
_____
_____

Stress levels at home
1 2 3 4 5
6 7 8 9 10

Stress levels at work
1 2 3 4 5
6 7 8 9 10

Daily Chronic Pain Tracker

Date:

Weather
Temp:
Condition:
Humidity:

My Symptoms
_____
_____
_____
_____

How well did you sleep?
1 2 3 4 5 6 7 8 9 10

How was your pain today?
1 2 3 4 5 6 7 8 9 10

How was your fatigue today?
1 2 3 4 5 6 7 8 9 10

How was your brain fog today?
1 2 3 4 5 6 7 8 9 10

How was your mood today?
1 2 3 4 5 6 7 8 9 10

Food Tracker
Breakfast
_____
_____
_____

Lunch
_____
_____
_____

Dinner
_____
_____
_____
_____

Snacks/Drinks
_____
_____

Code & Color in your Pain

[ ]	*Shooting*
[ ]	*Stabbing*
[ ]	*Burning*
[ ]	*Numbness*
[ ]	*Aching*
[ ]	*Pins & Needles*
[ ]	*Other*

Medication

Supplements

Vitamins

NOTES
_____
_____
_____
_____
_____
_____
_____
_____
_____
_____
_____
_____
_____

Stress levels at home
1 2 3 4 5
6 7 8 9 10

Stress levels at work
1 2 3 4 5
6 7 8 9 10

Daily Chronic Pain Tracker

Date:

Weather
Temp:
Condition:
Humidity:

My Symptoms
_____
_____
_____
_____

How well did you sleep?
1 2 3 4 5 6 7 8 9 10

How was your pain today?
1 2 3 4 5 6 7 8 9 10

How was your fatigue today?
1 2 3 4 5 6 7 8 9 10

How was your brain fog today?
1 2 3 4 5 6 7 8 9 10

How was your mood today?
1 2 3 4 5 6 7 8 9 10

Code & Color in your Pain

☐	Shooting
☐	Stabbing
☐	Burning
☐	Numbness
☐	Aching
☐	Pins & Needles
☐	Other

NOTES
_____
_____
_____
_____
_____
_____
_____
_____
_____
_____
_____
_____
_____
_____

Stress levels at home
1 2 3 4 5
6 7 8 9 10

Stress levels at work
1 2 3 4 5
6 7 8 9 10

Food Tracker

Breakfast
_____
_____
_____

Lunch
_____
_____
_____

Dinner
_____
_____
_____
_____

Snacks/Drinks
_____
_____
_____

Medication

Supplements

Vitamins

Daily Chronic Pain Tracker

Date:

Weather
Temp:
Condition:
Humidity:

My Symptoms
_____
_____
_____
_____

How well did you sleep?
1 2 3 4 5 6 7 8 9 10

How was your pain today?
1 2 3 4 5 6 7 8 9 10

How was your fatigue today?
1 2 3 4 5 6 7 8 9 10

How was your brain fog today?
1 2 3 4 5 6 7 8 9 10

How was your mood today?
1 2 3 4 5 6 7 8 9 10

Food Tracker
Breakfast
_____
_____
_____

Lunch
_____
_____
_____

Dinner
_____
_____
_____
_____

Snacks/Drinks
_____
_____
_____

Code & Color in your Pain

[ ] Shooting
[ ] Stabbing
[ ] Burning
[ ] Numbness
[ ] Aching
[ ] Pins & Needles
[ ] Other

Medication

NOTES
_____
_____
_____
_____
_____
_____
_____
_____
_____
_____
_____
_____

Stress levels at home
1 2 3 4 5
6 7 8 9 10

Stress levels at work
1 2 3 4 5
6 7 8 9 10

Supplements

Vitamins

Daily Chronic Pain Tracker

Date:

Weather
Temp:
Condition:
Humidity:

My Symptoms
_____
_____
_____
_____

How well did you sleep?
1 2 3 4 5 6 7 8 9 10

How was your pain today?
1 2 3 4 5 6 7 8 9 10

How was your fatigue today?
1 2 3 4 5 6 7 8 9 10

How was your brain fog today?
1 2 3 4 5 6 7 8 9 10

How was your mood today?
1 2 3 4 5 6 7 8 9 10

Food Tracker

Breakfast _____
_____
_____

Lunch _____
_____
_____

Dinner
_____
_____
_____
_____

Snacks/Drinks
_____
_____
_____

Code & Color in your Pain

[ ] *Shooting*
[ ] *Stabbing*
[ ] *Burning*
[ ] *Numbness*
[ ] *Aching*
[ ] *Pins & Needles*
[ ] *Other*

Medication

Supplements

Vitamins

NOTES
_____
_____
_____
_____
_____
_____
_____
_____
_____
_____
_____

Stress levels at home
1 2 3 4 5
6 7 8 9 10

Stress levels at work
1 2 3 4 5
6 7 8 9 10

Daily Chronic Pain Tracker

Date:

Weather
Temp:
Condition:
Humidity:

My Symptoms
_____
_____
_____

How well did you sleep?
1 2 3 4 5 6 7 8 9 10

How was your pain today?
1 2 3 4 5 6 7 8 9 10

How was your fatigue today?
1 2 3 4 5 6 7 8 9 10

How was your brain fog today?
1 2 3 4 5 6 7 8 9 10

How was your mood today?
1 2 3 4 5 6 7 8 9 10

Food Tracker

Breakfast
_____
_____
_____

Lunch
_____
_____

Dinner
_____
_____
_____
_____

Snacks/Drinks
_____
_____
_____

Code & Color in your Pain

☐	Shooting
☐	Stabbing
☐	Burning
☐	Numbness
☐	Aching
☐	Pins & Needles
☐	Other

Medication

Supplements

Vitamins

NOTES
_____
_____
_____
_____
_____
_____
_____
_____
_____
_____
_____
_____

Stress levels at home
1 2 3 4 5
6 7 8 9 10

Stress levels at work
1 2 3 4 5
6 7 8 9 10

Daily Chronic Pain Tracker

Date:

Weather
Temp:
Condition:
Humidity:

My Symptoms
_____
_____
_____
_____

How well did you sleep?
1 2 3 4 5 6 7 8 9 10

How was your pain today?
1 2 3 4 5 6 7 8 9 10

How was your fatigue today?
1 2 3 4 5 6 7 8 9 10

How was your brain fog today?
1 2 3 4 5 6 7 8 9 10

How was your mood today?
1 2 3 4 5 6 7 8 9 10

Food Tracker

Breakfast
_____
_____
_____

Lunch
_____
_____
_____

Dinner
_____
_____
_____
_____

Snacks/Drinks
_____
_____
_____

Code & Color in your Pain

[ ] Shooting
[ ] Stabbing
[ ] Burning
[ ] Numbness
[ ] Aching
[ ] Pins & Needles
[ ] Other

Medication

Supplements

Vitamins

NOTES
_____
_____
_____
_____
_____
_____
_____
_____
_____
_____
_____
_____

Stress levels at home
1 2 3 4 5
6 7 8 9 10

Stress levels at work
1 2 3 4 5
6 7 8 9 10

Daily Chronic Pain Tracker

Date:

Weather
Temp:
Condition:
Humidity:

My Symptoms
_____
_____
_____
_____

How well did you sleep?
1 2 3 4 5 6 7 8 9 10

How was your pain today?
1 2 3 4 5 6 7 8 9 10

How was your fatigue today?
1 2 3 4 5 6 7 8 9 10

How was your brain fog today?
1 2 3 4 5 6 7 8 9 10

How was your mood today?
1 2 3 4 5 6 7 8 9 10

Food Tracker
Breakfast
_____
_____
_____

Lunch
_____
_____
_____

Dinner
_____
_____
_____
_____

Snacks/Drinks
_____
_____
_____

Code & Color in your Pain

☐	Shooting
☐	Stabbing
☐	Burning
☐	Numbness
☐	Aching
☐	Pins & Needles
☐	Other

Medication

Supplements

Vitamins

NOTES
_____
_____
_____
_____
_____
_____
_____
_____
_____
_____
_____
_____
_____

Stress levels at home
1 2 3 4 5
6 7 8 9 10

Stress levels at work
1 2 3 4 5
6 7 8 9 10

Daily Chronic Pain Tracker

Date:

Weather

Temp:

Condition:

Humidity:

My Symptoms
_____
_____
_____
_____

How well did you sleep?

1 2 3 4 5 6 7 8 9 10

How was your pain today?

1 2 3 4 5 6 7 8 9 10

How was your fatigue today?

1 2 3 4 5 6 7 8 9 10

How was your brain fog today?

1 2 3 4 5 6 7 8 9 10

How was your mood today?

1 2 3 4 5 6 7 8 9 10

Food Tracker

Breakfast _____
_____
_____
_____

Lunch _____
_____
_____
_____

Dinner _____
_____
_____
_____
_____

Code & Color
in your Pain

[ ]	Shooting
[ ]	Stabbing
[ ]	Burning
[ ]	Numbness
[ ]	Aching
[ ]	Pins & Needles
[ ]	Other

Snacks/Drinks
_____
_____
_____

Medication

NOTES
_____
_____
_____
_____
_____
_____
_____
_____
_____
_____
_____

Supplements

Vitamins

Stress levels at home

1 2 3 4 5
6 7 8 9 10

Stress levels at work

1 2 3 4 5
6 7 8 9 10

Daily Chronic Pain Tracker

Date:

Weather
Temp:
Condition:
Humidity:

My Symptoms
_____
_____
_____
_____

How well did you sleep?
1 2 3 4 5 6 7 8 9 10

How was your pain today?
1 2 3 4 5 6 7 8 9 10

How was your fatigue today?
1 2 3 4 5 6 7 8 9 10

How was your brain fog today?
1 2 3 4 5 6 7 8 9 10

How was your mood today?
1 2 3 4 5 6 7 8 9 10

Food Tracker
Breakfast
_____
_____
_____

Lunch
_____
_____
_____

Dinner
_____
_____
_____
_____

Snacks/Drinks
_____
_____
_____

Code & Color in your Pain

[ ] *Shooting*
[ ] *Stabbing*
[ ] *Burning*
[ ] *Numbness*
[ ] *Aching*
[ ] *Pins & Needles*
[ ] *Other*

Medication

NOTES
_____
_____
_____
_____
_____
_____
_____
_____
_____
_____
_____
_____
_____

Supplements

Vitamins

Stress levels at home
1 2 3 4 5
6 7 8 9 10

Stress levels at work
1 2 3 4 5
6 7 8 9 10

Daily Chronic Pain Tracker

Date:

Weather
Temp:
Condition:
Humidity:

My Symptoms
_____
_____
_____

How well did you sleep?
1 2 3 4 5 6 7 8 9 10

How was your pain today?
1 2 3 4 5 6 7 8 9 10

How was your fatigue today?
1 2 3 4 5 6 7 8 9 10

How was your brain fog today?
1 2 3 4 5 6 7 8 9 10

How was your mood today?
1 2 3 4 5 6 7 8 9 10

Food Tracker
Breakfast
_____
_____
_____

Lunch
_____
_____
_____

Dinner
_____
_____
_____
_____

Code & Color in your Pain

| | Shooting |
| Stabbing |
| Burning |
| Numbness |
| Aching |
| Pins & Needles |
| Other |

Snacks/Drinks
_____
_____
_____

Medication

NOTES
_____
_____
_____
_____
_____
_____

Stress levels at home
1 2 3 4 5
6 7 8 9 10

Supplements

_____
_____
_____
_____
_____

Vitamins

Stress levels at work
1 2 3 4 5
6 7 8 9 10

_____
_____

Daily Chronic Pain Tracker

Date:

Weather

Temp:

Condition:

Humidity:

My Symptoms

_____
_____
_____
_____

How well did you sleep?
1 2 3 4 5 6 7 8 9 10

How was your pain today?
1 2 3 4 5 6 7 8 9 10

How was your fatigue today?
1 2 3 4 5 6 7 8 9 10

How was your brain fog today?
1 2 3 4 5 6 7 8 9 10

How was your mood today?
1 2 3 4 5 6 7 8 9 10

Food Tracker

Breakfast
_____
_____
_____

Lunch
_____
_____
_____

Dinner
_____
_____
_____
_____

Snacks/Drinks
_____
_____
_____

Code & Color in your Pain

☐	Shooting
☐	Stabbing
☐	Burning
☐	Numbness
☐	Aching
☐	Pins & Needles
☐	Other

Medication

Supplements

Vitamins

NOTES
_____
_____
_____
_____
_____
_____
_____
_____
_____
_____

Stress levels at home

1 2 3 4 5
6 7 8 9 10

Stress levels at work

1 2 3 4 5
6 7 8 9 10

Daily Chronic Pain Tracker

Date:

Weather

Temp:

Condition:

Humidity:

My Symptoms

_____
_____
_____
_____

How well did you sleep?
1 2 3 4 5 6 7 8 9 10

How was your pain today?
1 2 3 4 5 6 7 8 9 10

How was your fatigue today?
1 2 3 4 5 6 7 8 9 10

How was your brain fog today?
1 2 3 4 5 6 7 8 9 10

How was your mood today?
1 2 3 4 5 6 7 8 9 10

Food Tracker

Breakfast
_____
_____
_____

Lunch
_____
_____
_____

Dinner
_____
_____
_____

Snacks/Drinks
_____
_____
_____

Code & Color in your Pain

[ ] *Shooting*

[ ] *Stabbing*

[ ] *Burning*

[ ] *Numbness*

[ ] *Aching*

[ ] *Pins & Needles*

[ ] *Other*

Medication

Supplements

Vitamins

NOTES
_____
_____
_____
_____
_____
_____
_____
_____
_____
_____
_____
_____

Stress levels at home

1 2 3 4 5
6 7 8 9 10

Stress levels at work

1 2 3 4 5
6 7 8 9 10

Daily Chronic Pain Tracker

Date:

Weather
Temp:
Condition:
Humidity:

My Symptoms
_____
_____
_____
_____

How well did you sleep?
1 2 3 4 5 6 7 8 9 10

How was your pain today?
1 2 3 4 5 6 7 8 9 10

How was your fatigue today?
1 2 3 4 5 6 7 8 9 10

How was your brain fog today?
1 2 3 4 5 6 7 8 9 10

How was your mood today?
1 2 3 4 5 6 7 8 9 10

Food Tracker
Breakfast _____
_____
_____
_____

Lunch _____
_____
_____

Dinner
_____
_____
_____
_____

Snacks/Drinks
_____
_____
_____

Code & Color in your Pain

☐	*Shooting*
☐	*Stabbing*
☐	*Burning*
☐	*Numbness*
☐	*Aching*
☐	*Pins & Needles*
☐	*Other*

Medication

NOTES
_____
_____
_____
_____
_____
_____
_____
_____
_____
_____
_____
_____

Supplements

Vitamins

Stress levels at home
1 2 3 4 5
6 7 8 9 10

Stress levels at work
1 2 3 4 5
6 7 8 9 10

Daily Chronic Pain Tracker

Date:

Weather
Temp:
Condition:
Humidity:

My Symptoms
_____
_____
_____
_____

How well did you sleep?
1 2 3 4 5 6 7 8 9 10

How was your pain today?
1 2 3 4 5 6 7 8 9 10

How was your fatigue today?
1 2 3 4 5 6 7 8 9 10

How was your brain fog today?
1 2 3 4 5 6 7 8 9 10

How was your mood today?
1 2 3 4 5 6 7 8 9 10

Food Tracker
Breakfast
_____
_____
_____

Lunch
_____
_____
_____

Dinner
_____
_____
_____
_____

Snacks/Drinks
_____
_____
_____

Code & Color in your Pain

[ ] Shooting
[ ] Stabbing
[ ] Burning
[ ] Numbness
[ ] Aching
[ ] Pins & Needles
[ ] Other

Medication

Supplements

Vitamins

NOTES
_____
_____
_____
_____
_____
_____
_____
_____
_____
_____
_____
_____
_____

Stress levels at home
1 2 3 4 5
6 7 8 9 10

Stress levels at work
1 2 3 4 5
6 7 8 9 10

Daily Chronic Pain Tracker

Date:

Weather

Temp:

Condition:

Humidity:

My Symptoms
_____
_____
_____

How well did you sleep?
1 2 3 4 5 6 7 8 9 10

How was your pain today?
1 2 3 4 5 6 7 8 9 10

How was your fatigue today?
1 2 3 4 5 6 7 8 9 10

How was your brain fog today?
1 2 3 4 5 6 7 8 9 10

How was your mood today?
1 2 3 4 5 6 7 8 9 10

Food Tracker

Breakfast
_____
_____
_____

Lunch
_____
_____
_____

Dinner
_____
_____
_____
_____

Snacks/Drinks
_____
_____
_____

Code & Color in your Pain

☐	*Shooting*
☐	*Stabbing*
☐	*Burning*
☐	*Numbness*
☐	*Aching*
☐	*Pins & Needles*
☐	*Other*

Medication

Supplements

Vitamins

NOTES
_____
_____
_____
_____
_____
_____
_____
_____
_____
_____
_____

Stress levels at home
1 2 3 4 5
6 7 8 9 10

Stress levels at work
1 2 3 4 5
6 7 8 9 10

Daily Chronic Pain Tracker

Date:

Weather
Temp:
Condition:
Humidity:

My Symptoms
_____
_____
_____
_____

How well did you sleep?
1 2 3 4 5 6 7 8 9 10

How was your pain today?
1 2 3 4 5 6 7 8 9 10

How was your fatigue today?
1 2 3 4 5 6 7 8 9 10

How was your brain fog today?
1 2 3 4 5 6 7 8 9 10

How was your mood today?
1 2 3 4 5 6 7 8 9 10

Food Tracker
Breakfast
_____
_____
_____

Lunch
_____
_____

Dinner
_____
_____
_____
_____

Snacks/Drinks
_____
_____
_____

Code & Color in your Pain

☐ Shooting
☐ Stabbing
☐ Burning
☐ Numbness
☐ Aching
☐ Pins & Needles
☐ Other

Medication

Supplements

Vitamins

NOTES
_____
_____
_____
_____
_____
_____
_____
_____
_____
_____
_____

Stress levels at home
1 2 3 4 5
6 7 8 9 10

Stress levels at work
1 2 3 4 5
6 7 8 9 10

Daily Chronic Pain Tracker

Date:

Weather
Temp:
Condition:
Humidity:

My Symptoms
_____
_____
_____

How well did you sleep?
1 2 3 4 5 6 7 8 9 10

How was your pain today?
1 2 3 4 5 6 7 8 9 10

How was your fatigue today?
1 2 3 4 5 6 7 8 9 10

How was your brain fog today?
1 2 3 4 5 6 7 8 9 10

How was your mood today?
1 2 3 4 5 6 7 8 9 10

Food Tracker
Breakfast _____
_____
_____

Lunch _____
_____
_____

Dinner _____
_____
_____
_____

Snacks/Drinks
_____
_____
_____

Code & Color in your Pain

[ ] Shooting
[ ] Stabbing
[ ] Burning
[ ] Numbness
[ ] Aching
[ ] Pins & Needles
[ ] Other

Medication

NOTES
_____
_____
_____
_____
_____
_____
_____
_____
_____
_____
_____
_____
_____

Supplements

Vitamins

Stress levels at home
1 2 3 4 5
6 7 8 9 10

Stress levels at work
1 2 3 4 5
6 7 8 9 10

Daily Chronic Pain Tracker

Date:

Weather
Temp:
Condition:
Humidity:

My Symptoms
_____
_____
_____

How well did you sleep?
1 2 3 4 5 6 7 8 9 10

How was your pain today?
1 2 3 4 5 6 7 8 9 10

How was your fatigue today?
1 2 3 4 5 6 7 8 9 10

How was your brain fog today?
1 2 3 4 5 6 7 8 9 10

How was your mood today?
1 2 3 4 5 6 7 8 9 10

Food Tracker
Breakfast _____
_____
_____
_____

Lunch _____
_____
_____
_____

Dinner _____
_____
_____
_____

Code & Color in your Pain

Shooting _____
Stabbing _____
Burning
Numbness
Aching
Pins & Needles
Other

Snacks/Drinks
_____
_____
_____

Medication

NOTES

_____
_____
_____
_____
_____
_____
_____
_____
_____
_____
_____
_____
_____
_____

Supplements

Vitamins

Stress levels at home
1 2 3 4 5
6 7 8 9 10

Stress levels at work
1 2 3 4 5
6 7 8 9 10

Daily Chronic Pain Tracker

Date:

Weather
Temp:
Condition:
Humidity:

My Symptoms
_____
_____
_____
_____

How well did you sleep?
1 2 3 4 5 6 7 8 9 10

How was your pain today?
1 2 3 4 5 6 7 8 9 10

How was your fatigue today?
1 2 3 4 5 6 7 8 9 10

How was your brain fog today?
1 2 3 4 5 6 7 8 9 10

How was your mood today?
1 2 3 4 5 6 7 8 9 10

Food Tracker
Breakfast
_____
_____
_____

Lunch
_____
_____
_____

Dinner
_____
_____
_____
_____

Snacks/Drinks
_____
_____
_____

Code & Color in your Pain

☐	Shooting
☐	Stabbing
☐	Burning
☐	Numbness
☐	Aching
☐	Pins & Needles
☐	Other

Medication

NOTES
_____
_____
_____
_____
_____
_____
_____
_____
_____
_____
_____
_____

Supplements

Vitamins

Stress levels at home
1 2 3 4 5
6 7 8 9 10

Stress levels at work
1 2 3 4 5
6 7 8 9 10

Daily Chronic Pain Tracker

Date:

Weather
Temp:
Condition:
Humidity:

My Symptoms
_____
_____
_____
_____

How well did you sleep?
1 2 3 4 5 6 7 8 9 10

How was your pain today?
1 2 3 4 5 6 7 8 9 10

How was your fatigue today?
1 2 3 4 5 6 7 8 9 10

How was your brain fog today?
1 2 3 4 5 6 7 8 9 10

How was your mood today?
1 2 3 4 5 6 7 8 9 10

Food Tracker
Breakfast
_____
_____

Lunch
_____
_____
_____

Dinner
_____
_____
_____
_____

Code & Color in your Pain

☐	*Shooting*
☐	*Stabbing*
☐	*Burning*
☐	*Numbness*
☐	*Aching*
☐	*Pins & Needles*
☐	*Other*

Snacks/Drinks
_____
_____
_____

Medication

Supplements

Vitamins

NOTES
_____
_____
_____
_____
_____
_____
_____
_____
_____
_____
_____
_____

Stress levels at home
1 2 3 4 5
6 7 8 9 10

Stress levels at work
1 2 3 4 5
6 7 8 9 10

Daily Chronic Pain Tracker

Date:

Weather

Temp:

Condition:

Humidity:

My Symptoms

_____
_____
_____
_____

How well did you sleep?
1 2 3 4 5 6 7 8 9 10

How was your pain today?
1 2 3 4 5 6 7 8 9 10

How was your fatigue today?
1 2 3 4 5 6 7 8 9 10

How was your brain fog today?
1 2 3 4 5 6 7 8 9 10

How was your mood today?
1 2 3 4 5 6 7 8 9 10

Food Tracker

Breakfast
_____
_____
_____

Lunch
_____
_____
_____

Dinner
_____
_____
_____
_____

Snacks/Drinks
_____
_____

Code & Color in your Pain

[ ] Shooting

[ ] Stabbing

[ ] Burning

[ ] Numbness

[ ] Aching

[ ] Pins & Needles

[ ] Other

Medication

NOTES

_____
_____
_____
_____
_____
_____
_____
_____
_____
_____

Supplements

Vitamins

Stress levels at home

1 2 3 4 5
6 7 8 9 10

Stress levels at work

1 2 3 4 5
6 7 8 9 10

Daily Chronic Pain Tracker

Date:

Weather
Temp:
Condition:
Humidity:

How well did you sleep?
1 2 3 4 5 6 7 8 9 10

How was your pain today?
1 2 3 4 5 6 7 8 9 10

How was your fatigue today?
1 2 3 4 5 6 7 8 9 10

My Symptoms
_____
_____
_____
_____

How was your brain fog today?
1 2 3 4 5 6 7 8 9 10

How was your mood today?
1 2 3 4 5 6 7 8 9 10

Food Tracker

Breakfast _____
_____
_____

Lunch _____
_____
_____

Dinner _____
_____
_____
_____
_____

Snacks/Drinks _____
_____
_____

Code & Color in your Pain

[____]	Shooting
[____]	Stabbing
[____]	Burning
[____]	Numbness
[____]	Aching
[____]	Pins & Needles
[____]	Other

Medication

Supplements

Vitamins

NOTES
_____
_____
_____
_____
_____
_____
_____
_____
_____
_____
_____
_____
_____

Stress levels at home
1 2 3 4 5
6 7 8 9 10

Stress levels at work
1 2 3 4 5
6 7 8 9 10

Daily Chronic Pain Tracker

Date:

Weather
Temp:
Condition:
Humidity:

My Symptoms
_____
_____
_____

How well did you sleep?
1 2 3 4 5 6 7 8 9 10

How was your pain today?
1 2 3 4 5 6 7 8 9 10

How was your fatigue today?
1 2 3 4 5 6 7 8 9 10

How was your brain fog today?
1 2 3 4 5 6 7 8 9 10

How was your mood today?
1 2 3 4 5 6 7 8 9 10

Food Tracker
Breakfast
_____
_____
_____

Lunch
_____
_____
_____

Dinner
_____
_____
_____
_____

Snacks/Drinks
_____
_____
_____

Code & Color in your Pain

[ ] Shooting
[ ] Stabbing
[ ] Burning
[ ] Numbness
[ ] Aching
[ ] Pins & Needles
[ ] Other

Medication

NOTES
_____
_____
_____
_____
_____
_____
_____
_____
_____
_____
_____
_____

Supplements

Vitamins

Stress levels at home
1 2 3 4 5
6 7 8 9 10

Stress levels at work
1 2 3 4 5
6 7 8 9 10

Daily Chronic Pain Tracker

Date:

Weather
Temp:
Condition:
Humidity:

My Symptoms
_____
_____
_____
_____

How well did you sleep?
1 2 3 4 5 6 7 8 9 10

How was your pain today?
1 2 3 4 5 6 7 8 9 10

How was your fatigue today?
1 2 3 4 5 6 7 8 9 10

How was your brain fog today?
1 2 3 4 5 6 7 8 9 10

How was your mood today?
1 2 3 4 5 6 7 8 9 10

Food Tracker

Breakfast _____
_____
_____

Lunch _____
_____
_____

Dinner _____
_____
_____
_____

Snacks/Drinks _____
_____
_____

Code & Color in your Pain

[ ] Shooting _____
[ ] Stabbing _____
[ ] Burning
[ ] Numbness
[ ] Aching
[ ] Pins & Needles
[ ] Other

Medication

NOTES
_____
_____
_____
_____
_____
_____
_____
_____
_____
_____
_____
_____
_____

Supplements

Vitamins

Stress levels at home
1 2 3 4 5
6 7 8 9 10

Stress levels at work
1 2 3 4 5
6 7 8 9 10

Daily Chronic Pain Tracker

Date:

Weather

Temp:

Condition:

Humidity:

My Symptoms

_____
_____
_____
_____

How well did you sleep?
1 2 3 4 5 6 7 8 9 10

How was your pain today?
1 2 3 4 5 6 7 8 9 10

How was your fatigue today?
1 2 3 4 5 6 7 8 9 10

How was your brain fog today?
1 2 3 4 5 6 7 8 9 10

How was your mood today?
1 2 3 4 5 6 7 8 9 10

Code & Color in your Pain

[ ] Shooting _____
[ ] Stabbing _____
[ ] Burning
[ ] Numbness
[ ] Aching
[ ] Pins & Needles
[ ] Other

NOTES
_____
_____
_____
_____
_____
_____
_____
_____
_____
_____
_____
_____

Stress levels at home

1 2 3 4 5
6 7 8 9 10

Stress levels at work

1 2 3 4 5
6 7 8 9 10

Food Tracker

Breakfast
_____
_____
_____

Lunch
_____
_____

Dinner
_____
_____
_____
_____

Snacks/Drinks
_____
_____

Medication

Supplements

Vitamins

Daily Chronic Pain Tracker

Date:

Weather

Temp:

Condition:

Humidity:

My Symptoms
_____
_____
_____
_____

How well did you sleep?
1 2 3 4 5 6 7 8 9 10

How was your pain today?
1 2 3 4 5 6 7 8 9 10

How was your fatigue today?
1 2 3 4 5 6 7 8 9 10

How was your brain fog today?
1 2 3 4 5 6 7 8 9 10

How was your mood today?
1 2 3 4 5 6 7 8 9 10

Food Tracker

Breakfast
_____
_____
_____

Lunch
_____
_____

Dinner
_____
_____
_____
_____

Snacks/Drinks
_____
_____
_____

Code & Color in your Pain

Shooting

Stabbing

Burning

Numbness

Aching

Pins & Needles

Other

Medication

Supplements

Vitamins

NOTES
_____
_____
_____
_____
_____
_____
_____
_____
_____
_____
_____

Stress levels at home
1 2 3 4 5
6 7 8 9 10

Stress levels at work
1 2 3 4 5
6 7 8 9 10

Daily Chronic Pain Tracker

Date:

Weather
Temp:
Condition:
Humidity:

My Symptoms
_____
_____
_____
_____

How well did you sleep?
1 2 3 4 5 6 7 8 9 10

How was your pain today?
1 2 3 4 5 6 7 8 9 10

How was your fatigue today?
1 2 3 4 5 6 7 8 9 10

How was your brain fog today?
1 2 3 4 5 6 7 8 9 10

How was your mood today?
1 2 3 4 5 6 7 8 9 10

Food Tracker
Breakfast _____
_____
_____
_____

Lunch _____
_____
_____

Dinner _____
_____
_____
_____
_____

Snacks/Drinks
_____
_____
_____

Code & Color in your Pain

[ ] Shooting
[ ] Stabbing
[ ] Burning
[ ] Numbness
[ ] Aching
[ ] Pins & Needles
[ ] Other

Medication

NOTES
_____
_____
_____
_____
_____
_____
_____
_____
_____
_____
_____
_____
_____

Supplements

Vitamins

Stress levels at home
1 2 3 4 5
6 7 8 9 10

Stress levels at work
1 2 3 4 5
6 7 8 9 10

Daily Chronic Pain Tracker

Date:

Weather
Temp:
Condition:
Humidity:

My Symptoms
_____
_____
_____
_____

How well did you sleep?
1 2 3 4 5 6 7 8 9 10

How was your pain today?
1 2 3 4 5 6 7 8 9 10

How was your fatigue today?
1 2 3 4 5 6 7 8 9 10

How was your brain fog today?
1 2 3 4 5 6 7 8 9 10

How was your mood today?
1 2 3 4 5 6 7 8 9 10

Food Tracker
Breakfast
_____
_____
_____

Lunch
_____
_____
_____

Dinner
_____
_____
_____
_____

Snacks/Drinks
_____
_____
_____

Code & Color in your Pain

▢ Shooting _____
▢ Stabbing _____
▢ Burning
▢ Numbness
▢ Aching
▢ Pins & Needles
▢ Other

Medication

NOTES
_____
_____
_____
_____
_____
_____
_____
_____
_____
_____
_____
_____
_____
_____
_____
_____

Stress levels at home
1 2 3 4 5
6 7 8 9 10

Stress levels at work
1 2 3 4 5
6 7 8 9 10

Supplements

Vitamins

Daily Chronic Pain Tracker

Date:

Weather

Temp:

Condition:

Humidity:

My Symptoms

_____

_____

_____

_____

How well did you sleep?
1 2 3 4 5 6 7 8 9 10

How was your pain today?
1 2 3 4 5 6 7 8 9 10

How was your fatigue today?
1 2 3 4 5 6 7 8 9 10

How was your brain fog today?
1 2 3 4 5 6 7 8 9 10

How was your mood today?
1 2 3 4 5 6 7 8 9 10

Food Tracker

Breakfast _____

_____

_____

Lunch _____

_____

_____

Dinner _____

_____

_____

_____

Snacks/Drinks

_____

_____

Code & Color in your Pain

[ ] Shooting

[ ] Stabbing

[ ] Burning

[ ] Numbness

[ ] Aching

[ ] Pins & Needles

[ ] Other

Medication

Supplements

Vitamins

NOTES

_____

_____

_____

_____

_____

_____

_____

_____

_____

_____

_____

_____

Stress levels at home

1 2 3 4 5

6 7 8 9 10

Stress levels at work

1 2 3 4 5

6 7 8 9 10

Daily Chronic Pain Tracker

Date:

Weather
Temp:
Condition:
Humidity:

My Symptoms
_____
_____
_____
_____

How well did you sleep?
1 2 3 4 5 6 7 8 9 10

How was your pain today?
1 2 3 4 5 6 7 8 9 10

How was your fatigue today?
1 2 3 4 5 6 7 8 9 10

How was your brain fog today?
1 2 3 4 5 6 7 8 9 10

How was your mood today?
1 2 3 4 5 6 7 8 9 10

Food Tracker

Breakfast _____
_____
_____
_____

Lunch
_____
_____
_____

Dinner
_____
_____
_____
_____

Snacks/Drinks
_____
_____
_____

Code & Color in your Pain

[   ] *Shooting* _____
[   ] *Stabbing* _____
[   ] *Burning*
[   ] *Numbness*
[   ] *Aching*
[   ] *Pins & Needles*
[   ] *Other*

Medication

Supplements

Vitamins

NOTES
_____
_____
_____
_____
_____
_____
_____
_____
_____
_____
_____
_____

Stress levels at home
1 2 3 4 5
6 7 8 9 10

Stress levels at work
1 2 3 4 5
6 7 8 9 10

Daily Chronic Pain Tracker

Date:

Weather
Temp:
Condition:
Humidity:

My Symptoms
_____
_____
_____

How well did you sleep?
1 2 3 4 5 6 7 8 9 10

How was your pain today?
1 2 3 4 5 6 7 8 9 10

How was your fatigue today?
1 2 3 4 5 6 7 8 9 10

How was your brain fog today?
1 2 3 4 5 6 7 8 9 10

How was your mood today?
1 2 3 4 5 6 7 8 9 10

Food Tracker
Breakfast
_____
_____
_____

Lunch
_____
_____

Dinner
_____
_____
_____
_____

Snacks/Drinks
_____
_____

Code & Color in your Pain

[ ] Shooting
[ ] Stabbing
[ ] Burning
[ ] Numbness
[ ] Aching
[ ] Pins & Needles
[ ] Other

Medication

Supplements

Vitamins

NOTES
_____
_____
_____
_____
_____
_____
_____
_____
_____
_____
_____
_____

Stress levels at home
1 2 3 4 5
6 7 8 9 10

Stress levels at work
1 2 3 4 5
6 7 8 9 10

Daily Chronic Pain Tracker

Date:

Weather
Temp:
Condition:
Humidity:

My Symptoms
_____
_____
_____
_____

How well did you sleep?
1 2 3 4 5 6 7 8 9 10

How was your pain today?
1 2 3 4 5 6 7 8 9 10

How was your fatigue today?
1 2 3 4 5 6 7 8 9 10

How was your brain fog today?
1 2 3 4 5 6 7 8 9 10

How was your mood today?
1 2 3 4 5 6 7 8 9 10

Food Tracker
Breakfast _____
_____
_____
Lunch _____
_____
_____
Dinner _____
_____
_____
_____
_____
Snacks/Drinks
_____
_____
_____

Code & Color in your Pain

- [ ] Shooting
- [ ] Stabbing
- [ ] Burning
- [ ] Numbness
- [ ] Aching
- [ ] Pins & Needles
- [ ] Other

Medication

Supplements

Vitamins

NOTES
_____
_____
_____
_____
_____
_____
_____
_____
_____
_____
_____
_____

Stress levels at home
1 2 3 4 5
6 7 8 9 10

Stress levels at work
1 2 3 4 5
6 7 8 9 10

Daily Chronic Pain Tracker

Date:

Weather
Temp:
Condition:
Humidity:

My Symptoms
_____
_____
_____
_____

How well did you sleep?
1 2 3 4 5 6 7 8 9 10

How was your pain today?
1 2 3 4 5 6 7 8 9 10

How was your fatigue today?
1 2 3 4 5 6 7 8 9 10

How was your brain fog today?
1 2 3 4 5 6 7 8 9 10

How was your mood today?
1 2 3 4 5 6 7 8 9 10

Food Tracker
Breakfast
_____
_____
_____

Lunch
_____
_____

Dinner
_____
_____
_____

Snacks/Drinks
_____
_____

Code & Color in your Pain

[ ]	Shooting
[ ]	Stabbing
[ ]	Burning
[ ]	Numbness
[ ]	Aching
[ ]	Pins & Needles
[ ]	Other

NOTES
_____
_____
_____
_____
_____
_____
_____
_____
_____
_____
_____
_____
_____
_____

Medication

Supplements

Vitamins

Stress levels at home
1 2 3 4 5
6 7 8 9 10

Stress levels at work
1 2 3 4 5
6 7 8 9 10

Daily Chronic Pain Tracker

Date:

Weather
Temp:
Condition:
Humidity:

My Symptoms
_____
_____
_____
_____

How well did you sleep?
1 2 3 4 5 6 7 8 9 10

How was your pain today?
1 2 3 4 5 6 7 8 9 10

How was your fatigue today?
1 2 3 4 5 6 7 8 9 10

How was your brain fog today?
1 2 3 4 5 6 7 8 9 10

How was your mood today?
1 2 3 4 5 6 7 8 9 10

Food Tracker
Breakfast _____
_____
_____

Lunch _____
_____
_____

Dinner _____
_____
_____
_____

Snacks/Drinks _____
_____
_____

Code & Color in your Pain

Shooting
Stabbing
Burning
Numbness
Aching
Pins & Needles
Other

Medication

Supplements

Vitamins

NOTES
_____
_____
_____
_____
_____
_____
_____
_____
_____
_____
_____
_____

Stress levels at home
1 2 3 4 5
6 7 8 9 10

Stress levels at work
1 2 3 4 5
6 7 8 9 10

Daily Chronic Pain Tracker

Date:

Weather
Temp:
Condition:
Humidity:

My Symptoms
_____
_____
_____
_____

How well did you sleep?
1 2 3 4 5 6 7 8 9 10

How was your pain today?
1 2 3 4 5 6 7 8 9 10

How was your fatigue today?
1 2 3 4 5 6 7 8 9 10

How was your brain fog today?
1 2 3 4 5 6 7 8 9 10

How was your mood today?
1 2 3 4 5 6 7 8 9 10

Food Tracker
Breakfast
_____
_____
_____

Lunch
_____
_____

Dinner
_____
_____
_____
_____

Snacks/Drinks
_____
_____
_____

Code & Color in your Pain

[ ] Shooting
[ ] Stabbing
[ ] Burning
[ ] Numbness
[ ] Aching
[ ] Pins & Needles
[ ] Other

NOTES
_____
_____
_____
_____
_____
_____
_____
_____
_____
_____
_____
_____
_____

Stress levels at home
1 2 3 4 5
6 7 8 9 10

Stress levels at work
1 2 3 4 5
6 7 8 9 10

Medication

Supplements

Vitamins

Daily Chronic Pain Tracker

Date:

Weather
Temp:
Condition:
Humidity:

My Symptoms
_____
_____
_____

How well did you sleep?
1 2 3 4 5 6 7 8 9 10

How was your pain today?
1 2 3 4 5 6 7 8 9 10

How was your fatigue today?
1 2 3 4 5 6 7 8 9 10

How was your brain fog today?
1 2 3 4 5 6 7 8 9 10

How was your mood today?
1 2 3 4 5 6 7 8 9 10

Food Tracker
Breakfast
_____
_____

Lunch
_____
_____
_____

Dinner
_____
_____
_____
_____

Snacks/Drinks
_____
_____
_____

Code & Color in your Pain

[ ] Shooting
[ ] Stabbing
[ ] Burning
[ ] Numbness
[ ] Aching
[ ] Pins & Needles
[ ] Other

Medication

Supplements

Vitamins

NOTES
_____
_____
_____
_____
_____
_____
_____
_____
_____
_____
_____

Stress levels at home
1 2 3 4 5
6 7 8 9 10

Stress levels at work
1 2 3 4 5
6 7 8 9 10

Daily Chronic Pain Tracker

Date:

Weather
Temp:
Condition:
Humidity:

My Symptoms
_____
_____
_____
_____

How well did you sleep?
1 2 3 4 5 6 7 8 9 10

How was your pain today?
1 2 3 4 5 6 7 8 9 10

How was your fatigue today?
1 2 3 4 5 6 7 8 9 10

How was your brain fog today?
1 2 3 4 5 6 7 8 9 10

How was your mood today?
1 2 3 4 5 6 7 8 9 10

Food Tracker
Breakfast
_____
_____
_____

Lunch
_____
_____
_____

Dinner
_____
_____
_____

Snacks/Drinks
_____
_____

Code & Color in your Pain

☐ Shooting
☐ Stabbing
☐ Burning
☐ Numbness
☐ Aching
☐ Pins & Needles
☐ Other

Medication

NOTES
_____
_____
_____
_____
_____
_____
_____
_____
_____
_____
_____
_____
_____
_____

Supplements

Stress levels at home
1 2 3 4 5
6 7 8 9 10

Stress levels at work
1 2 3 4 5
6 7 8 9 10

Vitamins

Daily Chronic Pain Tracker

Date:

Weather
Temp:
Condition:
Humidity:

My Symptoms
_____
_____
_____
_____

How well did you sleep?
1 2 3 4 5 6 7 8 9 10

How was your pain today?
1 2 3 4 5 6 7 8 9 10

How was your fatigue today?
1 2 3 4 5 6 7 8 9 10

How was your brain fog today?
1 2 3 4 5 6 7 8 9 10

How was your mood today?
1 2 3 4 5 6 7 8 9 10

Food Tracker
Breakfast
_____
_____
_____

Lunch
_____
_____
_____

Dinner
_____
_____
_____
_____

Code & Color in your Pain

☐ Shooting
☐ Stabbing
☐ Burning
☐ Numbness
☐ Aching
☐ Pins & Needles
☐ Other

Snacks/Drinks
_____
_____
_____

Medication

NOTES
_____
_____
_____
_____
_____
_____
_____

Supplements

Stress levels at home
1 2 3 4 5
6 7 8 9 10

Stress levels at work
1 2 3 4 5
6 7 8 9 10

_____
_____
_____
_____
_____
_____

Vitamins

Daily Chronic Pain Tracker

Date:

Weather
Temp:
Condition:
Humidity:

My Symptoms
_____
_____
_____

How well did you sleep?
1 2 3 4 5 6 7 8 9 10

How was your pain today?
1 2 3 4 5 6 7 8 9 10

How was your fatigue today?
1 2 3 4 5 6 7 8 9 10

How was your brain fog today?
1 2 3 4 5 6 7 8 9 10

How was your mood today?
1 2 3 4 5 6 7 8 9 10

Food Tracker
Breakfast
_____
_____
_____

Lunch
_____
_____
_____

Dinner
_____
_____
_____
_____

Snacks/Drinks
_____
_____

Code & Color in your Pain

[ ] Shooting
[ ] Stabbing
[ ] Burning
[ ] Numbness
[ ] Aching
[ ] Pins & Needles
[ ] Other

Medication

NOTES
_____
_____
_____
_____
_____
_____
_____
_____
_____
_____
_____
_____
_____

Supplements

Vitamins

Stress levels at home
1 2 3 4 5
6 7 8 9 10

Stress levels at work
1 2 3 4 5
6 7 8 9 10

Daily Chronic Pain Tracker

Date:

Weather
Temp:
Condition:
Humidity:

My Symptoms
_____
_____
_____
_____

How well did you sleep?
1 2 3 4 5 6 7 8 9 10

How was your pain today?
1 2 3 4 5 6 7 8 9 10

How was your fatigue today?
1 2 3 4 5 6 7 8 9 10

How was your brain fog today?
1 2 3 4 5 6 7 8 9 10

How was your mood today?
1 2 3 4 5 6 7 8 9 10

Food Tracker
Breakfast _____
_____
_____
_____

Lunch
_____
_____
_____
_____

Dinner
_____
_____
_____
_____
_____

Snacks/Drinks
_____
_____
_____

Code & Color in your Pain

[ ] *Shooting* _____
[ ] *Stabbing* _____
[ ] *Burning*
[ ] *Numbness*
[ ] *Aching*
[ ] *Pins & Needles*
[ ] *Other*

Medication

NOTES
_____
_____
_____
_____
_____
_____
_____

Supplements

_____
_____
_____
_____
_____
_____

Vitamins

Stress levels at home
1 2 3 4 5
6 7 8 9 10

Stress levels at work
1 2 3 4 5
6 7 8 9 10

Daily Chronic Pain Tracker

Date:

Weather
Temp:
Condition:
Humidity:

My Symptoms
_____
_____
_____
_____

How well did you sleep?
1 2 3 4 5 6 7 8 9 10

How was your pain today?
1 2 3 4 5 6 7 8 9 10

How was your fatigue today?
1 2 3 4 5 6 7 8 9 10

How was your brain fog today?
1 2 3 4 5 6 7 8 9 10

How was your mood today?
1 2 3 4 5 6 7 8 9 10

Food Tracker

Breakfast
_____
_____
_____

Lunch
_____
_____
_____

Dinner
_____
_____
_____
_____

Snacks/Drinks
_____
_____

Code & Color in your Pain

[ ]	Shooting
[ ]	Stabbing
[ ]	Burning
[ ]	Numbness
[ ]	Aching
[ ]	Pins & Needles
[ ]	Other

Medication

Supplements

Vitamins

NOTES
_____
_____
_____
_____
_____
_____
_____
_____
_____
_____
_____
_____

Stress levels at home
1 2 3 4 5
6 7 8 9 10

Stress levels at work
1 2 3 4 5
6 7 8 9 10

Daily Chronic Pain Tracker

Date:

Weather
Temp:
Condition:
Humidity:

My Symptoms
_____
_____
_____
_____

How well did you sleep?
1 2 3 4 5 6 7 8 9 10

How was your pain today?
1 2 3 4 5 6 7 8 9 10

How was your fatigue today?
1 2 3 4 5 6 7 8 9 10

How was your brain fog today?
1 2 3 4 5 6 7 8 9 10

How was your mood today?
1 2 3 4 5 6 7 8 9 10

Food Tracker
Breakfast
_____
_____
_____

Lunch
_____
_____
_____

Dinner
_____
_____
_____
_____
_____

Snacks/Drinks
_____
_____
_____

Code & Color in your Pain

☐ *Shooting*
☐ *Stabbing*
☐ *Burning*
☐ *Numbness*
☐ *Aching*
☐ *Pins & Needles*
☐ *Other*

Medication

Supplements

Vitamins

NOTES
_____
_____
_____
_____
_____
_____
_____
_____
_____
_____
_____

Stress levels at home
1 2 3 4 5
6 7 8 9 10

Stress levels at work
1 2 3 4 5
6 7 8 9 10

Daily Chronic Pain Tracker

Date:

Weather
Temp:
Condition:
Humidity:

My Symptoms
_____
_____
_____

How well did you sleep?
1 2 3 4 5 6 7 8 9 10

How was your pain today?
1 2 3 4 5 6 7 8 9 10

How was your fatigue today?
1 2 3 4 5 6 7 8 9 10

How was your brain fog today?
1 2 3 4 5 6 7 8 9 10

How was your mood today?
1 2 3 4 5 6 7 8 9 10

Food Tracker
Breakfast
_____
_____
_____

Lunch
_____
_____
_____

Dinner
_____
_____
_____
_____

Code & Color in your Pain

[ ] Shooting
[ ] Stabbing
[ ] Burning
[ ] Numbness
[ ] Aching
[ ] Pins & Needles
[ ] Other

Snacks/Drinks
_____
_____
_____

Medication

NOTES
_____
_____
_____
_____
_____
_____
_____
_____
_____
_____
_____
_____
_____

Supplements

Vitamins

Stress levels at home
1 2 3 4 5
6 7 8 9 10

Stress levels at work
1 2 3 4 5
6 7 8 9 10

Daily Chronic Pain Tracker

Date:

Weather
Temp:
Condition:
Humidity:

My Symptoms
_____
_____
_____
_____

How well did you sleep?
1 2 3 4 5 6 7 8 9 10

How was your pain today?
1 2 3 4 5 6 7 8 9 10

How was your fatigue today?
1 2 3 4 5 6 7 8 9 10

How was your brain fog today?
1 2 3 4 5 6 7 8 9 10

How was your mood today?
1 2 3 4 5 6 7 8 9 10

Food Tracker
Breakfast _____
_____
_____
_____

Lunch _____
_____
_____

Dinner _____
_____
_____
_____

Snacks/Drinks _____
_____
_____

Code & Color in your Pain

☐ Shooting
☐ Stabbing
☐ Burning
☐ Numbness
☐ Aching
☐ Pins & Needles
☐ Other

Medication

Supplements

Vitamins

NOTES
_____
_____
_____
_____
_____
_____
_____
_____
_____
_____
_____
_____

Stress levels at home
1 2 3 4 5
6 7 8 9 10

Stress levels at work
1 2 3 4 5
6 7 8 9 10

Daily Chronic Pain Tracker

Date:

Weather
Temp:
Condition:
Humidity:

My Symptoms
_____
_____
_____
_____

How well did you sleep?
1 2 3 4 5 6 7 8 9 10

How was your pain today?
1 2 3 4 5 6 7 8 9 10

How was your fatigue today?
1 2 3 4 5 6 7 8 9 10

How was your brain fog today?
1 2 3 4 5 6 7 8 9 10

How was your mood today?
1 2 3 4 5 6 7 8 9 10

Code & Color in your Pain

[ ] Shooting
[ ] Stabbing
[ ] Burning
[ ] Numbness
[ ] Aching
[ ] Pins & Needles
[ ] Other

NOTES
_____
_____
_____
_____
_____
_____
_____
_____
_____
_____
_____

Food Tracker
Breakfast
_____
_____
_____

Lunch
_____
_____
_____

Dinner
_____
_____
_____
_____

Snacks/Drinks
_____
_____

Medication

Supplements

Vitamins

Stress levels at home
1 2 3 4 5
6 7 8 9 10

Stress levels at work
1 2 3 4 5
6 7 8 9 10

Daily Chronic Pain Tracker

Date:

Weather
Temp:
Condition:
Humidity:

My Symptoms
_____
_____
_____
_____

How well did you sleep?
1 2 3 4 5 6 7 8 9 10

How was your pain today?
1 2 3 4 5 6 7 8 9 10

How was your fatigue today?
1 2 3 4 5 6 7 8 9 10

How was your brain fog today?
1 2 3 4 5 6 7 8 9 10

How was your mood today?
1 2 3 4 5 6 7 8 9 10

Food Tracker
Breakfast _____
_____
_____

Lunch _____
_____
_____

Dinner _____
_____
_____
_____

Snacks/Drinks _____
_____
_____

Code & Color in your Pain

☐ Shooting
☐ Stabbing
☐ Burning
☐ Numbness
☐ Aching
☐ Pins & Needles
☐ Other

Medication

Supplements

Vitamins

NOTES
_____
_____
_____
_____
_____
_____
_____
_____
_____
_____
_____
_____

Stress levels at home
1 2 3 4 5
6 7 8 9 10

Stress levels at work
1 2 3 4 5
6 7 8 9 10

Daily Chronic Pain Tracker

Date:

Weather
Temp:
Condition:
Humidity:

My Symptoms
_____
_____
_____

How well did you sleep?
1 2 3 4 5 6 7 8 9 10

How was your pain today?
1 2 3 4 5 6 7 8 9 10

How was your fatigue today?
1 2 3 4 5 6 7 8 9 10

How was your brain fog today?
1 2 3 4 5 6 7 8 9 10

How was your mood today?
1 2 3 4 5 6 7 8 9 10

Food Tracker
Breakfast
_____
_____
_____

Lunch
_____
_____
_____

Dinner
_____
_____
_____
_____

Snacks/Drinks
_____
_____

Code & Color in your Pain

☐ Shooting
☐ Stabbing
☐ Burning
☐ Numbness
☐ Aching
☐ Pins & Needles
☐ Other

Medication

NOTES
_____
_____
_____
_____
_____
_____
_____
_____
_____
_____
_____
_____
_____
_____
_____

Supplements

Vitamins

Stress levels at home
1 2 3 4 5
6 7 8 9 10

Stress levels at work
1 2 3 4 5
6 7 8 9 10

Daily Chronic Pain Tracker

Date:

Weather
Temp:
Condition:
Humidity:

My Symptoms
_____
_____
_____

How well did you sleep?
1 2 3 4 5 6 7 8 9 10

How was your pain today?
1 2 3 4 5 6 7 8 9 10

How was your fatigue today?
1 2 3 4 5 6 7 8 9 10

How was your brain fog today?
1 2 3 4 5 6 7 8 9 10

How was your mood today?
1 2 3 4 5 6 7 8 9 10

Food Tracker
Breakfast
_____
_____
_____

Lunch
_____
_____
_____

Dinner
_____
_____
_____

Snacks/Drinks
_____
_____

Code & Color in your Pain

[ ] Shooting
[ ] Stabbing
[ ] Burning
[ ] Numbness
[ ] Aching
[ ] Pins & Needles
[ ] Other

Medication

NOTES
_____
_____
_____
_____
_____
_____
_____
_____
_____
_____

Supplements

Vitamins

Stress levels at home
1 2 3 4 5
6 7 8 9 10

Stress levels at work
1 2 3 4 5
6 7 8 9 10

Daily Chronic Pain Tracker

Date:

Weather
Temp:
Condition:
Humidity:

My Symptoms
_____
_____
_____

How well did you sleep?
1 2 3 4 5 6 7 8 9 10

How was your pain today?
1 2 3 4 5 6 7 8 9 10

How was your fatigue today?
1 2 3 4 5 6 7 8 9 10

How was your brain fog today?
1 2 3 4 5 6 7 8 9 10

How was your mood today?
1 2 3 4 5 6 7 8 9 10

Food Tracker
Breakfast
_____
_____
_____

Lunch
_____
_____
_____

Dinner
_____
_____
_____
_____

Snacks/Drinks
_____
_____
_____

Code & Color
in your Pain

[   ] Shooting
[   ] Stabbing
[   ] Burning
[   ] Numbness
[   ] Aching
[   ] Pins & Needles
[   ] Other

Medication

Supplements

Vitamins

NOTES
_____
_____
_____
_____
_____
_____
_____
_____
_____
_____

Stress levels at home
1 2 3 4 5
6 7 8 9 10

Stress levels at work
1 2 3 4 5
6 7 8 9 10

Daily Chronic Pain Tracker

Date:

Weather

Temp:

Condition:

Humidity:

My Symptoms

_____
_____
_____
_____

How well did you sleep?

1 2 3 4 5 6 7 8 9 10

How was your pain today?

1 2 3 4 5 6 7 8 9 10

How was your fatigue today?

1 2 3 4 5 6 7 8 9 10

How was your brain fog today?

1 2 3 4 5 6 7 8 9 10

How was your mood today?

1 2 3 4 5 6 7 8 9 10

Food Tracker

Breakfast
_____
_____
_____

Lunch
_____
_____
_____

Dinner
_____
_____
_____
_____

Snacks/Drinks
_____
_____
_____

Code & Color in your Pain

[ ] Shooting

[ ] Stabbing

[ ] Burning

[ ] Numbness

[ ] Aching

[ ] Pins & Needles

[ ] Other

NOTES

_____
_____
_____
_____
_____
_____
_____
_____
_____
_____
_____
_____

Medication

Supplements

Vitamins

Stress levels at home

1 2 3 4 5
6 7 8 9 10

Stress levels at work

1 2 3 4 5
6 7 8 9 10

Daily Chronic Pain Tracker

Date:

Weather

Temp:

Condition:

Humidity:

My Symptoms

_____

_____

_____

_____

How well did you sleep?

1 2 3 4 5 6 7 8 9 10

How was your pain today?

1 2 3 4 5 6 7 8 9 10

How was your fatigue today?

1 2 3 4 5 6 7 8 9 10

How was your brain fog today?

1 2 3 4 5 6 7 8 9 10

How was your mood today?

1 2 3 4 5 6 7 8 9 10

Food Tracker

Breakfast

_____

_____

Lunch

_____

_____

Dinner

_____

_____

_____

Code & Color in your Pain

[ ] Shooting

[ ] Stabbing

[ ] Burning

[ ] Numbness

[ ] Aching

[ ] Pins & Needles

[ ] Other

Snacks/Drinks

_____

_____

NOTES

_____

_____

_____

_____

_____

_____

_____

_____

_____

_____

_____

_____

Medication

Supplements

Vitamins

Stress levels at home

1 2 3 4 5

6 7 8 9 10

Stress levels at work

1 2 3 4 5

6 7 8 9 10

Daily Chronic Pain Tracker

Date:

Weather
Temp:
Condition:
Humidity:

My Symptoms
_____
_____
_____
_____

How well did you sleep?
1 2 3 4 5 6 7 8 9 10

How was your pain today?
1 2 3 4 5 6 7 8 9 10

How was your fatigue today?
1 2 3 4 5 6 7 8 9 10

How was your brain fog today?
1 2 3 4 5 6 7 8 9 10

How was your mood today?
1 2 3 4 5 6 7 8 9 10

Food Tracker
Breakfast _____
_____
_____

Lunch _____
_____
_____

Dinner _____
_____
_____
_____

Snacks/Drinks
_____
_____

Code & Color in your Pain

[ ] Shooting
[ ] Stabbing
[ ] Burning
[ ] Numbness
[ ] Aching
[ ] Pins & Needles
[ ] Other

Medication

NOTES
_____
_____
_____
_____
_____
_____

Supplements

Stress levels at home
1 2 3 4 5
6 7 8 9 10

Stress levels at work
1 2 3 4 5
6 7 8 9 10

Vitamins

Daily Chronic Pain Tracker

Date:

Weather
Temp:
Condition:
Humidity:

My Symptoms
_____
_____
_____

How well did you sleep?
1 2 3 4 5 6 7 8 9 10

How was your pain today?
1 2 3 4 5 6 7 8 9 10

How was your fatigue today?
1 2 3 4 5 6 7 8 9 10

How was your brain fog today?
1 2 3 4 5 6 7 8 9 10

How was your mood today?
1 2 3 4 5 6 7 8 9 10

Food Tracker
Breakfast
_____
_____
_____

Lunch
_____
_____
_____

Dinner
_____
_____
_____
_____

Snacks/Drinks
_____
_____

Code & Color
in your Pain

[ ] Shooting
[ ] Stabbing
[ ] Burning
[ ] Numbness
[ ] Aching
[ ] Pins & Needles
[ ] Other

Medication

Supplements

Vitamins

NOTES
_____
_____
_____
_____
_____
_____
_____
_____
_____
_____
_____
_____
_____
_____
_____

Stress levels at home
1 2 3 4 5
6 7 8 9 10

Stress levels at work
1 2 3 4 5
6 7 8 9 10

Daily Chronic Pain Tracker

Date:

How well did you sleep?
1 2 3 4 5 6 7 8 9 10

Weather
Temp:

How was your pain today?
1 2 3 4 5 6 7 8 9 10

Condition:

Humidity:

How was your fatigue today?
1 2 3 4 5 6 7 8 9 10

My Symptoms

How was your brain fog today?
1 2 3 4 5 6 7 8 9 10

_____

_____

How was your mood today?
1 2 3 4 5 6 7 8 9 10

_____

Food Tracker

Breakfast
_____
_____
_____

Lunch
_____
_____
_____

Dinner
_____
_____
_____

Code & Color in your Pain

[ ]	Shooting
[ ]	Stabbing
[ ]	Burning
[ ]	Numbness
[ ]	Aching
[ ]	Pins & Needles
[ ]	Other

Snacks/Drinks
_____
_____

Medication

NOTES

_____
_____
_____
_____
_____
_____
_____
_____

Supplements

Stress levels at home

1 2 3 4 5
6 7 8 9 10

Stress levels at work

1 2 3 4 5
6 7 8 9 10

Vitamins

Daily Chronic Pain Tracker

Date:

Weather

Temp:

Condition:

Humidity:

My Symptoms

_____

_____

_____

_____

How well did you sleep?
1 2 3 4 5 6 7 8 9 10

How was your pain today?
1 2 3 4 5 6 7 8 9 10

How was your fatigue today?
1 2 3 4 5 6 7 8 9 10

How was your brain fog today?
1 2 3 4 5 6 7 8 9 10

How was your mood today?
1 2 3 4 5 6 7 8 9 10

Food Tracker

Breakfast _____

_____

_____

Lunch _____

_____

_____

Dinner _____

_____

_____

_____

Snacks/Drinks

_____

_____

Code & Color in your Pain

	Shooting
	Stabbing
	Burning
	Numbness
	Aching
	Pins & Needles
	Other

Medication

NOTES

_____

_____

_____

_____

Stress levels at home

1 2 3 4 5
6 7 8 9 10

Stress levels at work

1 2 3 4 5
6 7 8 9 10

Supplements

Vitamins

Daily Chronic Pain Tracker

Date: _____

Weather
Temp: _____
Condition: _____
Humidity: _____

My Symptoms
_____
_____
_____
_____

How well did you sleep?
1 2 3 4 5 6 7 8 9 10

How was your pain today?
1 2 3 4 5 6 7 8 9 10

How was your fatigue today?
1 2 3 4 5 6 7 8 9 10

How was your brain fog today?
1 2 3 4 5 6 7 8 9 10

How was your mood today?
1 2 3 4 5 6 7 8 9 10

Code & Color in your Pain

[ ] Shooting
[ ] Stabbing
[ ] Burning
[ ] Numbness
[ ] Aching
[ ] Pins & Needles
[ ] Other

NOTES
_____
_____
_____
_____
_____
_____
_____
_____
_____
_____
_____
_____

Stress levels at home
1 2 3 4 5
6 7 8 9 10

Stress levels at work
1 2 3 4 5
6 7 8 9 10

Food Tracker
Breakfast
_____
_____

Lunch
_____
_____

Dinner
_____
_____
_____

Snacks/Drinks
_____
_____

Medication

Supplements

Vitamins

Daily Chronic Pain Tracker

Date:

Weather

Temp:

Condition:

Humidity:

My Symptoms

_____

_____

_____

_____

How well did you sleep?

1 2 3 4 5 6 7 8 9 10

How was your pain today?

1 2 3 4 5 6 7 8 9 10

How was your fatigue today?

1 2 3 4 5 6 7 8 9 10

How was your brain fog today?

1 2 3 4 5 6 7 8 9 10

How was your mood today?

1 2 3 4 5 6 7 8 9 10

Code & Color in your Pain

[ ]	Shooting
[ ]	Stabbing
[ ]	Burning
[ ]	Numbness
[ ]	Aching
[ ]	Pins & Needles
[ ]	Other

NOTES

_____

_____

_____

_____

_____

_____

_____

_____

_____

_____

_____

Food Tracker

Breakfast

_____

_____

_____

Lunch

_____

_____

_____

Dinner

_____

_____

_____

_____

Snacks/Drinks

_____

_____

_____

Medication

Supplements

Vitamins

Stress levels at home

1 2 3 4 5

6 7 8 9 10

Stress levels at work

1 2 3 4 5

6 7 8 9 10

Daily Chronic Pain Tracker

Date:

Weather
Temp:
Condition:
Humidity:

My Symptoms
_____
_____
_____

How well did you sleep?
1 2 3 4 5 6 7 8 9 10

How was your pain today?
1 2 3 4 5 6 7 8 9 10

How was your fatigue today?
1 2 3 4 5 6 7 8 9 10

How was your brain fog today?
1 2 3 4 5 6 7 8 9 10

How was your mood today?
1 2 3 4 5 6 7 8 9 10

Food Tracker

Breakfast
_____
_____
_____

Lunch
_____
_____

Dinner
_____
_____
_____

Snacks/Drinks
_____
_____

Code & Color in your Pain

[ ] Shooting
[ ] Stabbing
[ ] Burning
[ ] Numbness
[ ] Aching
[ ] Pins & Needles
[ ] Other

Medication

Supplements

Vitamins

NOTES
_____
_____
_____
_____
_____
_____
_____
_____
_____
_____
_____

Stress levels at home
1 2 3 4 5
6 7 8 9 10

Stress levels at work
1 2 3 4 5
6 7 8 9 10

Daily Chronic Pain Tracker

Date:

Weather
Temp:
Condition:
Humidity:

My Symptoms
_____
_____
_____
_____

How well did you sleep?
1 2 3 4 5 6 7 8 9 10

How was your pain today?
1 2 3 4 5 6 7 8 9 10

How was your fatigue today?
1 2 3 4 5 6 7 8 9 10

How was your brain fog today?
1 2 3 4 5 6 7 8 9 10

How was your mood today?
1 2 3 4 5 6 7 8 9 10

Food Tracker
Breakfast
_____
_____
_____

Lunch
_____
_____
_____

Dinner
_____
_____
_____
_____

Snacks/Drinks
_____
_____

Code & Color in your Pain

Shooting

Stabbing

Burning

Numbness

Aching

Pins & Needles

Other

Medication

NOTES
_____
_____
_____
_____
_____
_____
_____
_____
_____
_____
_____
_____

Supplements

Vitamins

Stress levels at home
1 2 3 4 5
6 7 8 9 10

Stress levels at work
1 2 3 4 5
6 7 8 9 10

Daily Chronic Pain Tracker

Date:

Weather
Temp:
Condition:
Humidity:

My Symptoms
_____
_____
_____

How well did you sleep?
1 2 3 4 5 6 7 8 9 10

How was your pain today?
1 2 3 4 5 6 7 8 9 10

How was your fatigue today?
1 2 3 4 5 6 7 8 9 10

How was your brain fog today?
1 2 3 4 5 6 7 8 9 10

How was your mood today?
1 2 3 4 5 6 7 8 9 10

Food Tracker
Breakfast
_____
_____

Lunch
_____
_____

Dinner
_____
_____

Code & Color
in your Pain

[ ] Shooting
[ ] Stabbing
[ ] Burning
[ ] Numbness
[ ] Aching
[ ] Pins & Needles
[ ] Other

Snacks/Drinks
_____
_____

Medication

NOTES
_____
_____
_____
_____
_____
_____
_____
_____
_____

Stress levels at home
1 2 3 4 5
6 7 8 9 10

Stress levels at work
1 2 3 4 5
6 7 8 9 10

Supplements

Vitamins

Daily Chronic Pain Tracker

Date:

Weather
Temp:
Condition:
Humidity:

My Symptoms
_____
_____
_____
_____

How well did you sleep?
1 2 3 4 5 6 7 8 9 10

How was your pain today?
1 2 3 4 5 6 7 8 9 10

How was your fatigue today?
1 2 3 4 5 6 7 8 9 10

How was your brain fog today?
1 2 3 4 5 6 7 8 9 10

How was your mood today?
1 2 3 4 5 6 7 8 9 10

Food Tracker
Breakfast
_____
_____
_____

Lunch
_____
_____
_____

Dinner
_____
_____
_____
_____

Snacks/Drinks
_____
_____
_____

Code & Color in your Pain

[ ] Shooting
[ ] Stabbing
[ ] Burning
[ ] Numbness
[ ] Aching
[ ] Pins & Needles
[ ] Other

NOTES
_____
_____
_____
_____
_____
_____
_____
_____
_____
_____
_____
_____
_____
_____

Stress levels at home
1 2 3 4 5
6 7 8 9 10

Stress levels at work
1 2 3 4 5
6 7 8 9 10

Medication

Supplements

Vitamins

CPSIA information can be obtained
at www.ICGtesting.com
Printed in the USA
LVHW010024040422
715224LV00010B/453

9 781649 441560